An Easy Way
To Understand
Herpes

Herpes Simplex • Genital Herpes
Herpes Zoster (Shingles)

Also By Brian B Jacques

His very popular Series of Mini-Health Books includes:

- An Easy Way To Understanding Eczema and Psoriasis
- An Easy Way To Understand Stress and Depression
- An Easy Way To Understand Vitamins and Minerals
- An Easy Way To Understand Parasites, Worms, Candida, Constipation & Detoxing
- An Easy Way To Understand Crohn's Disease and IBD
- An Easy Way To Understand Body Building For Men And Women
- An Easy Way To Understand Alzheimer's Disease
- An Easy Way To Understand Herpes
- An Easy Way To Understand Parkinson's Disease
- An Easy Way To Understand Autism
- An Easy Way To Understand Fibromyalgia
- An Easy Way To Understand Your Body Systems
- An Easy Way To Understand Erectile Dysfunction
- An Easy Way To Understand Heart Disease, High Blood Pressure & Stroke
- An Easy Way To Understand Detoxing For Men & Women
- How To Lose Weight After 40
- How To Lose Weight And Maintain Your Ideal Weight Permanently
- Amino Acids & Enzymes—What Are They & Why Do You Need Them
- The Little A–Z Dictionary of Herbal Remedies
- The Magic Of Vitamins & Minerals
- Effective Methods To Stop Smoking
- Eat Wholefoods And Take Supplements—The Ultimate Lifestyle Guide
- Stress Busters Adult Coloring Book

All these books are available as Kindle Editions (available from the Kindle Store on Amazon.com, and other countries Amazon sites where the Kindle platform is supported.) Many of these books are also available for the Barnes and Noble "Nook". In addition, many of these titles are available as print editions from the Amazon website.

An Easy Way To Understand Herpes

Herpes Simplex • Genital Herpes Herpes Zoster (Shingles)

Brian B Jacques

Wisdom For Life Media

"Education is the kindling of a flame, not the filling of a vessel." —Socrates

Contents

Acknowledgment

To the many people I have come into contact with throughout my life, whose belief in me has made everything possible and worthwhile.

Brian B Jacques

1. So What is Herpes

Herpes is a virus which comes in various forms: The most common form is Herpes Simplex virus 1 (HSV-1) which is usually associated with cold sores around the mouth, nose and eyes. Herpes Simplex Virus 2 (HSV-2) which is referred to as genital herpes and then there is Varicella Zoster virus which is better known as chickenpox which affects children and young adults. This virus remains dormant in the body until a person gets older when it reappears as Herpes Zoster virus, which is probably better known as shingles.

Of the world population, it is estimated that over 50 percent of the white population, over 70 percent of the African American population and over 60 percent of the Japanese population have herpes.

Instances of herpes amongst the American population are on the increase, due in part to lax sexual attitudes and a lack of adequate protection when having sex.

Alarmingly, someone may not even know that they have the disease, unless there are visible signs. Another thing! Once you have herpes—then you have got it for life. There is no cure, and all that can be done is try and keep it in remission by taking medications prescribed by your doctor. In addition, you can make sure that your immune system is working at optimum efficiency, that you eat a healthy diet, and consider taking some vitamin and mineral supplements and herbal medicines which I discuss in this book.

In addition, a herpes infection can be extremely harmful to your overall good health, and it is also highly contagious. The caveat then is to learn all you can about the disease, and how you can protect yourself from getting infected.

What is Herpes Simplex Virus

Cold sores around the mouth, nose and eyes are the result of being infected with the herpes simplex virus (HSV-1). You may have been infected as a child when someone kissed you at a time when they had the virus in its infectious stage.

The virus then entered your mouth and found a "home" in a host cell—in all probability a nerve cell. The virus then ordered the DNA in the nerve cell to produce more viruses, which it was more than happy to do. You will have the herpes virus in your body for life, and any subsequent eruptions will normally appear at the same spot as the time before.

A cold sore usually starts as a tingling and burning sensation, this is followed by a series of blisters which are lumps filled with clear liquid. These blisters usually run together to form one big blister. This big blister burns and swells until it breaks open and forms a yellow crust and then fades away. The time line from start to finish is approximately 10 to 21 days. No scar is left behind.

Open ulcers are highly contagious. Don't touch it, and don't touch anyone else. Don't touch the sore and then rub your eyes, nose or genitals.

There are several drugs: Acyclovir, Famciclovir and Valacyclovir used to treat all strains of herpes—whether it is in the mouth, genitals or shingles. Acyclovir is available as a capsule, tablet or liquid. The liquid can be applied to the affected area and then the tablet can be taken orally. The other two medications are only available in tablet form. These drugs prevent the virus from reproducing.

Anesthetic ointments which contain Benzocaine can be applied directly to the sore to numb it enough so you can eat properly—but this won't speed healing.

There are however, various medicinal herbs that can offer some relief, and I have covered a few of these later in this book.

How Does Genital Herpes Differ

Genital herpes is different to cold sores. Genital herpes is mainly an adult infection caused by being infected with the herpes simplex virus type 2 (HSV-2). However, the virus can cause a re-occurrence on virtually any part of the skin or mucus membranes.

As mentioned previously, HSV-1 is usually characterized by cold sores around the mouth area, whilst HSV-2 (genital herpes) is characterized by clusters of small blisters which are filled with a clear fluid and have a reddish colored base, and they are usually located in the genital area—as the name suggests. Eventually the blisters burst which then leaves behind small, but very painful ulcers which usually heal within 10 to 21 days.

Now to add a bit of confusion! Statistics show that approximately 40 percent of people who have mouth sores actually have the herpes strain that affects the genitals. And, approximately 60 percent of the infections found in the genital area are in fact the herpes simplex type 1 strain that usually affects the mouth area.

Remember what I mentioned earlier—the infection can in fact appear anywhere on the skin or mucus membranes. Therefore you can get an infection on the lips, gums roof of the mouth, in the nostrils, on the fingers and around the eye area and on the eye lids.

To give you some idea of the numbers, roughly 90 percent of the world's population is infected with HSV-1. After the initial infection, the virus appears to remain dormant in the nerve cells in the majority of people. It can however, be reactivated, usually when the immune system is looking after other problems in the body, or when a person is under stress or is suffering from some other illness.

However, other factors can cause a re-occurrence including: spicy food, sunlight, the menstrual cycle, rainy days and fever.

One of the key issues in preventing a re-occurrence is to keep the immune system healthy.

2. Herpes Simplex Virus

Herpes simplex virus type I (HSV-1), often appears as ulcers or blisters around the mouth area when a person first comes into contact with the HSV-1 virus. The first attack may be quite severe, with subsequent outbreaks being quite mild. However, other people may have no symptoms at all.

After the first infection the virus becomes dormant in the nerve tissue of the face. In some individuals the virus reactivates itself at a later stage causing cold sores.

The blisters may appear within one to three weeks after first contact with the virus, and the infection may last up to three weeks. Indications that you may have the herpes virus include: itching, a burning sensation and/or a tingling sensation around the mouth area.

Before the blisters appear, you may have a fever, sore throat, swollen glands and/or pain while swallowing. The blisters may develop on your gums, lips, around or inside the mouth as well as the throat area.

There may be several blisters which spread to form one large blister. These blisters will be filled with a clear yellowish colored fluid which will often break open and start discharging. As the blister heals, it will form a yellow crust which eventually will fall off and pink colored healing skin will be revealed.

Herpes symptoms may be triggered by several causes including: hormonal changes, menstruation changes, being exposed to excessive sunshine which causes sunburn, having a fever and being under stress; all of these factors have an impact on the immune system which is the body's main line of defense in fighting infection.

If you suspect that you have a herpes infection then your doctor can perform a diagnosis by looking at your mouth area. Sometimes your doctor will take a sample of the sore and forward it to a laboratory for examination.

In many individuals, the infection will go away on its own without any treatment in one to two weeks. In some cases, your doctor can prescribe antiviral medication to alleviate the pain associated with your symptoms and help eradicate the infection sooner. Medications used to treat a mouth infection include: Acyclovir, Famciclovir and Valacyclovir.

These medications work best when taken at the first warning signs of an infection, before any blisters appear. If you are one of those individuals who have frequent herpes infections, then your doctor may advise you to take these medications on a continual basis.

Also, antiviral skin creams may also be applied. Unfortunately, these can be rather expensive and only shorten the outbreak by a small length of time.

You may wish to try some of the following to help you feel more comfortable during the period of the infection:

• Apply an ice pack or a warm washcloth to the sores to help ease the pain. But remember to discard the ice pack and washcloth after each use because it may carry some of the viral spores which have been shed, and if you use these items again, you may re-infect yourself.

• Wash the blisters with an antiseptic soap and water. This will help prevent spreading of the virus to other areas of the body.

• It is best to avoid hot, spicy foods, citrus fruits and hot beverages while you have the viral infection.

• If the infection is in your throat you can gargle with cool water and rinse with salt water.

• You can try a pain reliever such as Tylenol.

Complications can arise if you have a compromised immune system due to certain diseases such as HIV/AIDS, or you are taking immunosuppressant drugs after having transplant surgery.

A few suggestions to help prevent a recurrence of herpes simplex type I virus.

• Consider applying sunblock or lip balm containing zinc oxide to your lips before you go out into the sunshine.

• Try and avoid direct contact with someone who has herpes sores. And especially, do not kiss them.

• Always wash towels and other fabric items in hot boiling water after each use.

• You can help prevent spreading the sores to other parts of your body by always washing your hands after touching a cold sore, and by using a cotton-tip swab to apply herpes medication to a cold sore.

• Under no circumstances share drinking utensils, straws, lip balm, or any other item for that matter with a person who has mouth sores.

It is best not to indulge in oral sex if you have mouth sores, especially if you have blisters. If you do, you could spread the virus to the genitals, causing herpes simplex virus2 (genital herpes). Please understand that you can spread oral and genital herpes viruses even when you do not have "active" mouth sores or blisters.

3. Do I Have Genital Herpes Virus

It can be difficult to detect genital herpes. However, there are often visible signs that an infection is present.

Visible signs include red lumps in and/or around the genital area, usually commencing approximately two weeks after the initial exposure to the herpes virus. In some cases they may spread to the anus and/or surrounding skin areas. In some instances the infection will develop within the vagina and/or the urinary tract.

These lumps will turn into blisters and then sores. Usually these sores form a yellow crust and become itchy. After approximately 21 days the sores will disappear. An eruption can be a single sore or a multitude of sores. As genital herpes is incurable more eruptions will occur at different times throughout life.

Additional symptoms may accompany any genital herpes eruptions. These may include: a reddening and/or sudden dryness of the genital area; painful burning and/or an itching sensation in the genital area, discharge from the vagina, difficulty urinating, a headache, fever and/or swollen glands.

One of the problems is that the genital herpes virus can remain inactive in many individuals and never cause any problems. Additionally, they may never show any signs or symptoms of the condition. Unfortunately they are still able to spread the genital herpes virus to others. On many occasions symptoms of genital herpes are associated with other conditions such as yeast infections and urinary tract infections.

If you are concerned and think that you may have contracted the disease then it is best to see your doctor right away. Your doctor can usually do a visual diagnosis and a blood test and/or a viral culture can also be done to check for the virus. Only by having a proper analysis done can you be certain that you have a genital herpes infection.

Where did My Genital Herpes Infection Come From?

For many people being diagnosed with genital herpes comes as a shock. In some cases the diagnosis is possibly a confirmation of the suspicion that something was not right about their own health or how their partner was behaving.

Next, comes a period of blame and then self-recrimination. Living with herpes is something that may take a bit of getting used to, but it does not mean that this is the end of your life.

As mentioned above, a diagnosis of a genital herpes infection can be done with a blood test. If there are no active lesions then a person may be diagnosed through the presence of antibodies in the blood.

A more accurate diagnosis may be done by the physician taking the top off a scab, and taking a swab from the base of the lesion which is then sent to a lab where they can grow a viral culture. Extracting a swab from the lesion can be very painful for the patient.

HSV-2 is an adult infection in the genital area with the virus being dominant in the sacral nerve which is located at the base of the spine when it is not active.. Current studies for the Western world put the incidence of HSV-2 at around one in eight people, or approximately 12 percent of the population. Interestingly only approximately one in five of those with antibodies have been diagnosed.

To give you an illustration take a room containing 40 people, five of these people have HSV-2 but only one is aware that they are infected. Three of the five may have had an isolated symptom once or twice. This could have been so insignificant that they thought it was a pimple, boil or infected hair follicle. The final one of the five never had a symptom and may never do so. For this last one and the other three undiagnosed individuals, they are often accused of having the infection and saying nothing, or they are accused of infidelity by their partner.

Over the past few years there has been a lot of publicity concerning safe sex, and this has changed many people's sex practices, believing that only protective sex using a condom means safe sex. However, health experts now report that nearly half of the new herpes diagnosis performed in clinics has been confirmed as HSV-1 in the genital area. This could indicate a high incidence of oral sex being performed and as a result, HSV-1 which is usually associated with cold sores around the mouth area is being transmitted to the genital area. In addition HSV-2 which is normally associated with genital herpes is being found in the mouth.

There is one upside to this diagnosis in that where the herpes virus is in an unnatural environment: that is HSV-1 is in the genital area, and HSV-2 is in the mouth then the symptoms are less severe and happen less frequently.

Another misconception that many individuals have is assuming that they are not infectious during dormant periods. Studies show that even when a couple are discordant meaning that one is positive and the other is negative, and they take every precaution to reduce the risk of transmission, in a 12 month period the transmission rate is still 10 percent.

These couples used condoms during what they thought were dormant periods, and abstained from sex when the viral infection reoccurred. Interestingly, researchers report that if one partner has not been infected in a 10 year period, then it is unlikely that there will be infected in the future. It is theorized that they have acquired some immunity from getting the disease—some mechanism that has not yet been identified.

The first infection of HSV-2 can last for a period of 10 days. Symptoms will include: all the glands of the body will the swollen the person will experience influenza like symptoms, genital burning, itching, pain when urinating, or an inability to urinate.

Subsequent infections may be just as severe as the first infection, particularly if the immune system is compromised possibly because it is busy sorting out a problem in another part of the body. Subsequent recurrences of HSV-2 usually last for between five and 10 days.

As a HSV infection requires skin to skin contact and shedding of viral content, HSV-2 infections are usually confined to the genital area. Areas that are infected include the vulva and Labia in women and penis and scrotum in men. This is due to penetrative sex being in a localized area.

Where someone has been infected with HSV-1 in the genital area, the area is often larger and distribution of the infection is more extensive due to oral sex being performed. Both viruses may be treated with antiviral drugs.

As discussed earlier in this section each virus has its own host environment. For an individual who is infected with HSV-1 on the genitals, this will mean that future infections will be less severe, and in some instances may only reappear once or twice during their lifetime. If the infection is HSV-2 on the genitals, then recurrences can vary tremendously.

Re-occurring infections have a lot to do with the state of the immune system. If the body is under stress, the diet is inadequate, there is a lack of sleep, there are instances of sunburn and for women issues with their menstrual cycle, then during the first year of infection the number of recurrences may range from one to 12, with the average being around four to five. In subsequent years the immune system may improve, and in addition, the individual learns what will trigger re-occurrences and therefore will try to avoid them; as a result, re-occurrences of the infection may fall to as few as one or two per year.

Additionally as individual learns to better recognize the symptoms of an impending recurrence, they are in a better position to administer antiviral drugs earlier. This can significantly reduce the severity and length of the infection, and potentially can prevent an infection altogether. It is important for the individual to remember that even though they have avoided a recurrence, they are still shedding the virus and they are still potentially infectious to their partner.

One strategy is to take maintenance doses of antiviral drugs each day to reduce the number of recurrences. Statistics show that half of all individuals who follow this strategy have no re-occurrences in a 12 months period. When this strategy is discontinued for whatever reason then a re-occurrence will be experienced within approximately three weeks.

A small number of female patients have required this maintenance therapy with antiviral drugs continuously since they initially became available over 15 years ago. As recurrences reduce the number and severity, most individuals eventually come to terms with their viral infection. In some instances however this is not the case. Physicians report that they need to refer between 10 to 20 percent of their patients for further psychological counseling, even though they are highly experienced with the disease counseling needed with regard to this infection.

Ready access to information by individuals who are infected is of paramount importance. This can be obtained anonymously from the Internet. Support groups can also be found on the Internet as well as through local clinics and sexual health clinics. Although you will have the herpes virus for the rest of your life, with proper management and care it should not inhibit you from enjoying a loving and secure relationship as well as living a long and happy life.

How to Protect Yourself from Genital Herpes

As mentioned previously, genital herpes is a sexually transmitted disease. Sexual contact with an infected person can transmit the disease to you. Genital herpes re-occurrences are very painful and it can affect a relationship. So how do you protect yourself from getting infected?

For much of the time the herpes virus remains dormant. Now imagine that you have unprotected sex with someone who is in a dormant state; there is a possibility that you will get infected. Even worse, having protected sex with someone who has active genital herpes sores will increase your risk of becoming infected yourself. Now consider this; those who have been infected with the virus may be unaware that they have the virus; in which case they will unknowingly pass the virus on to you.

One of the things you can do to protect yourself from genital herpes is to avoid multiple partners. There is no way of knowing if one of your multiple partners has genital herpes. When you start a relationship with a new partner try to discreetly discover if they have any symptoms of genital herpes. This may sound like a sneaky thing to do but it is important that you protect yourself. It is best to avoid oral sex as this is unprotected sex.

If You Suffer from Herpes Rejection

If you have the herpes virus and are honest enough to tell the other person about it before you get involved sexually, and the other person rejects you as a result of your infection, then this can really knock your self-esteem and confidence. Each individual who is infected with the herpes virus will have to find their own way of dealing with it.

As a result of this rejection many people stop dating altogether, or they only date other people who also have herpes.

However, having a partner who also has herpes does not mean that you can now have unprotected sex. Indulging in unprotected sex with each other can make a herpes infection worse for one or both parties. It is called re-inoculation, and having this is not a good idea.

If you have the herpes virus it will make you more vulnerable to contracting other sexually transmitted diseases including HIV, cervical dysplasia and genital warts.

Experience shows that men are not always as protective of their sex partners concerning telling them that they have herpes as women are. It is important that men discuss with their potential female sex partners that they have herpes. A herpes infection is more devastating for a woman than it is for a man. In addition, it is much easier for a man to infect a woman than it is for a woman to infect a man.

Having herpes is a great test as to who might want you, and who might not. Any reasonable person would want to discuss the risks with someone who they thought was desirable before they knew you have herpes—and they may still think so afterwards—it will all depend on the person.

You can explain that you treat your herpes condition with medication and/or herbal medicine in addition to practicing safe sex with a condom, and use antiviral gel then this might reassure the person.

In many cases, fear is the great driver here, so you may have to accept rejection. And if you have been rejected then it is up to you how you handle it. At least you have been honest with the other person and as a result, you have nothing to feel guilty about. It could be that the other person was not really all that interested in you and this was as good a reason as any to end the relationship.

4. Herpes and other Medical Conditions

Eye Pain and Herpes

A herpes infection can be dangerous if it appears in or around the eye area (herpes keratitis). In some cases the infection can spread to one or both eyes. If this happens you may suffer pain, light sensitivity, liquid discharge as well as a gritty feeling in the eye. A herpes infection of the eye is one of the leading causes of blindness in the United States, as it causes scarring of the cornea.

The cornea—the clear outer lens of the eye, has a very thin outer skin that covers, and provides protection for the many sensitive nerves that reside within.

Should the cornea be damaged or become infected, then a crater which is really an ulcer will form. Because the nerves within the cornea become active, a lot of pain is generated.

If the ulcer is central in the eye area, then vision can be compromised, and should the ulcer penetrate to any depth then the cornea may be damaged. This is so serious that vision can be permanently damaged. If the virus gets lodged in the eye then it is probably there for life.

The condition may be cured with the proper treatment. However, if steroid ointments or drops are used, then this could permanently establish the virus, with the result that year of eye problems lie ahead.

Do you have a Bad Headache

Headaches are caused by all sorts of conditions in life from stress, worry, anxiety to getting bad tempered and irritable or having a bad cold or the flu. But there could be more to it than that. Take encephalitis for example, which is inflammation of the brain. This can cause a very severe headache as well as vomiting and a stiff neck and back. But what can cause this? The simple answer is usually an infection caused by a virus. And yes, you have probably guessed right. The herpes simplex or herpes zoster virus, or it could be polio viruses, echoviruses or coxsackie viruses.

Encephalitis is more often found in children rather than adults. It can occur due to a compromised immune system, by AIDS or by undergoing medical treatment for serious health conditions.

Herpes and Meningitis

A fever and a stiff neck in a child who has obvious signs of being ill can set alarm bells ringing that this could be a case of meningitis. What is meningitis? It is basically inflammation of the "meninges"— the membranes that cover the brain and spinal; cord.

The main cause of meningitis is a virus infection: usually herpes simplex, chickenpox, polio, mumps, echo, or coxsackie viruses.

It is best to take no chances with viral meningitis. It can be mild or more severe and in some cases can induce a coma. It is therefore important to seek immediate medical help.

Intercourse Pain

If genital or vaginal herpes causes you pain, then it is best to avoid having sex until the infection has cleared up. It is also advisable to use condoms at all times.

5. Here are Some Things That Will Help

Replace your toothbrush.

Your toothbrush is a great harborer of viruses and bacteria—and especially when you have a herpes infection. The virus can remain there for days, giving you a great re-infection when the current one has subsided. Therefore replace your toothbrush, or you could try dipping it in colloidal silver which is known to kill viruses.

Use small tubes of toothpaste.

How often do you touch the bristles in the toothbrush on the top of the toothpaste tube? Almost always I would suspect when you are getting the toothpaste out. Think of this! When you have a herpes infection, you then transfer the virus to the top of the toothpaste tube. Therefore if you use small tubes of toothpaste, then you will replace it more often and reduce the risk of re-infecting yourself.

Keep your toothpaste anywhere but in the bathroom.

Why? Well, the bathroom is usually moist—especially after taking a shower or a bath; then combine this with a wet toothbrush and you have an ideal environment for the herpes virus to remain active on your toothbrush for many more days. It is therefore best to keep it anywhere else but in the bathroom.

Towels.

Towels are carriers of disease—and should never be shared with anyone else. Ideally, they should be changed every day and the dirty ones put in the washing machine immediately and washed on the "hot" water cycle with an appropriate washing machine detergent. And this is especially important if you have a herpes re-occurrence, because you don't want to keep re-infecting yourself.

When you are outside in a sunny climate

Make sure you protect your lips from sunburn or wind exposure. This is something that is so easy to do with a protecting ointment, and it could save you from a herpes flare-up.

6. Eat a Healthy Diet

You can do this by eating a diet which is rich in antioxidant fruits and vegetables, making sure you get the omega 3 and omega 6 essential fatty acids; this can be achieved by eating oily fish such as salmon, tuna, mackerel and herrings (for omega 3), or supplementing with flaxseed oil which is rich in omega 3 and omega 6.

Further benefits can be obtained by cutting down on red meat and substituting for white meat such as chicken and turkey—but make sure the chicken and turkey come from an organic source, otherwise the white meat you eat could be loaded with growth promoters and hormones. Drink alcohol in moderation and only take medications when necessary.

And finally make sure you get some physical exercise. Exercise stimulates the immune system to produce white blood cells. These are the fighters which control infections in the body such as bacteria and viruses as well as other foreign invaders. Exercise is also good for your circulatory system which means your heart gets some exercise too. All the body systems are interlinked, so exercising will benefit your whole body.

Supplementing with the amino acid lysine can be a good idea too. Lysine helps inhibit the growth of the herpes simplex virus and as a result, reduces the number of outbreaks. Lysine also helps control the acid/alkaline balance in the body, and is one of the building blocks of blood antibodies.

Another important function it plays is in the absorption of calcium and the formation of collagen which is needed for bone, cartilage and the growth of connective tissue. Lysine needs the help of vitamin C before it can be utilized in the formation of collagen.

If vitamin C or protein is missing in the lysine supply cycle, then wounds will not heal properly and the body will be more susceptible to infection.

Good food sources of lysine include: beans, brewer's yeast, chicken, fish, milk and potatoes. Quite high doses of lysine are needed to make a significant difference—more than can be obtained from food. Therefore it is best to add a lysine supplement (take one or two 500 milligram tablets each day, depending on how severe the herpes infection is) which is available from health food stores or on the Internet.

Another amino acid is involved in herpes simplex infections too. This one is called arginine. The herpes simplex virus needs arginine to grow and develop.

As far as the virus is concerned, lysine and arginine look similar, so the idea is to trick the virus into using lysine instead of arginine.

Therefore restricting your dietary intake of arginine, and eliminating it altogether during an outbreak will be a good strategy to follow. Foods that are rich in arginine include: beer, cereals, chocolate, gelatin, peas, peanuts and raisins.

7. The Medications

Acyclovir

Acyclovir is prescribed to help reduce pain, speed up healing for mouth sores or blisters, for genital herpes, and for those who have an outbreak of the herpes zoster shingles) virus. This medications function is to stop the spread of the herpes virus within the body. Please note this medication does not cure genital herpes and will not stop the spread of the genital herpes virus to other people.

Acyclovir is available as a tablet, capsule or as a liquid by mouth. It can be taken with or without food two to five times a day for five to 10 days. It is best to start as soon as possible after your symptoms start. Take the medication as directed on the label and advised by your doctor.

You should take the medication until you have completed the prescription, even if your symptoms have disappeared. If you stop taking it too soon on miss doses, your infection may not be completely treated or may become more difficult to treat.

Famciclovir

Famciclovir is an antiviral medicine which is prescribed for people who have repeat outbreaks of herpes simplex 1—cold sores and do not have a compromised immune system. It is also used to treat outbreaks of genital herpes in individuals who do not have a compromised immune system. It is also prescribed to help prevent further outbreaks in the future. Famciclovir is also used to treat cases of herpes zoster (shingles).

This medication will not cure herpes infections and may not stop the spread of a herpes infection to other people. It is useful however, for reducing pain, burning sensations and tingling as well as helping sores to heal and preventing new sores from forming.

Famciclovir is available in tablet form to be taken by mouth with or without food. Follow the directions on the label and take it for the length of time advised by your doctor.

Valacyclovir

Valacyclovir is prescribed to treat genital herpes and herpes zoster (shingles) virus. It will not cure herpes infections but it does help decrease the pain and itching associated with these viruses as well as helping to heal sores and prevent new ones from forming.

Valacyclovir is available as a tablet to be taken by mouth. Follow the directions on the label and take it for the length of time advised by your doctor.

Even if your symptoms clear up, and you feel well, do not stop taking the medication without consulting your doctor first.

8. Alternatives to Medication

There are not a lot of medications that are available to treat a herpes infection. Basically it comes down to acyclovir, famciclovir, valacyclovir, butylated hydroxytoluene (BHT) and various creams. But there are quite a few medicinal herbs and also some vitamin and mineral supplements that you can consider. So here goes!

Medicinal Herbs for Herpes Simplex and Genital Herpes

Aloe Vera

Used in a gel form, aloe vera has been used for long periods as a medicinal and first aid treatment. The plants many soothing property are especially beneficial for burn victims as well as reducing inflammation and itching.

Aloe Vera can be used both internally (as a juice) and externally as a gel. It has tremendous healing properties when used on skin eruptions. It can also be combined with goldenseal to increase its healing properties.

Astragalus

Astragalus is used extensively in Traditional Chinese Medicine (TCM), and has been so used for centuries. Its prime use is to strengthen the immune system to fight off foreign invaders. It is especially useful in fighting colds and flu and in treating recurrent infections.

Chinese researchers has demonstrated its effectiveness in helping the body resist viral infections, especially in the lungs by increasing the production of interferon—an immune factor that prevents viral growth.

Black Walnut

Probably best known as an anti-parasitic and for eliminating worms. The black walnut tree produces fruit, not nuts as the name might suggest. The outer rind of these fruits contains a black colored tannin which has astringent properties. When this is applied topically it helps tone and heal inflamed tissues.

Burdock

Burdock is a very useful herb in the treatment of a herpes infection. Its insulin content helps heal herpes sores, and in addition, it has the ability to cleanse the blood of impurities and toxins.

Cat's Claw (Una de Gato)

A native species of the Peruvian rainforest, the native Indians make it into a tea to detoxify the body and strengthen the immune system. According to researchers, cat's claw helps counteract the effects of chemotherapy and radiotherapy in patients suffering from cancer. In fact, cat's claw is used extensively as a cancer treatment.

Cat's claw has also been shown to have excellent anti-viral properties to fight such viruses as herpes simplex and herpes zoster (shingles).

Colloidal Silver

Colloidal silver is an excellent antibiotic and can be used internally and externally. With the rise in bacterial organisms that are becoming resistant to antibiotic treatments, colloidal silver has no such problems in killing them. It has proved effective against many different bacterial, fungal and viral infections.

Used for hundreds of years as a medicinal, preserving and purifying agent, colloidal silver is now becoming well known as a treatment for many 21st century ailments. Pathogens are unable to formulate a resistance to colloidal silver. This is one of the reasons why it is so effective. In fact colloidal silver is effective in destroying over 650 disease causing organisms. It is a natural antiviral product.

Colloidal silver is very effective as a treatment for acne, ear, nose and throat infections, eczema, eye infections, herpes simplex type 1 and type 2, shingles, tonsillitis and viral warts. These are just a few of the many benefits that colloidal silver offers—there are many more.

When sourcing a colloidal silver product, it is important to make sure that there are no additives or fillers added; such as aluminium, lead or arsenic. Pure .999 ions silver diluted in deionized water which has been colloided is best.

Echinacea

The purple colored flowers of the Echinacea plant (a member of the daisy family) are a welcome addition to many gardens. Much research has been done on the benefits of Echinacea as an immune system strengthener. It is often taken at the first signs of a cold or flu and is extremely effective for this purpose.

Echinacea is an effective blood and lymph system cleanser, and in addition, when applied topically, it has excellent properties to clear skin conditions associated with viral infections such as herpes.

Echinacea contains a chemical called echinacein which protects body tissue against the hyaluronidase enzyme which many germs carry. Germs use this enzyme to penetrate body tissue and cause infections.

Echinacea is a useful topical treatment for herpes infections as it not only helps prevent germs from entering body tissue, but it also assists in encouraging new skin to knit together more quickly. It does this by encouraging cells to form new tissue (fibroblasts).

Garlic

Garlic is certainly versatile. Not only is it used in cooking, but it also has excellent health benefits as well. It helps protect against heart disease and stroke, it is also a natural antibiotic.

To get the antibiotic action working, an antibiotic element in the garlic clove called alliin has to be activated. To achieve this, the garlic clove must be crushed, sliced or bruised to help activate an enzyme allinase. When allinase and alliin come into contact with each other, another chemical called allicin is formed—and it is this later chemical which is the powerful antibiotic. Sounds a bit complicated doesn't it?

In one study, patients who took one clove of garlic each day for 3 months saw chronic herpes sores clear up.

Ginseng

Ginseng is not one herb but three: Korean ginseng, American ginseng and Siberian ginseng. Although the latter is not a true ginseng, it has similar properties to the other two.

All three contain several chemicals called ginsenosides which provide its therapeutic and healing actions. It is usually used as a tonic to increase stamina as well as to support the immune system and reduce cholesterol levels.

It has anti-clotting properties, thus helping to prevent blockages in arteries which could cause a heart attack or stroke. It also protects the liver from the harmful effects of drugs, alcohol, and other toxic substances.

It minimizes cell damage from radiation therapy, and for our topic in this book—herpes. In one study, ginseng's antiviral action eliminated chronic herpes sores. When the ginseng treatment was discontinued, the herpes sores returned.

Goldenseal

Goldenseal has been used for centuries by Native Americans to treat a variety of conditions, including healing cuts, wounds, improving appetite, for the relief of liver and stomach problems, and for repelling insects when mixed with bear grease.

Goldenseal helps heal damaged tissues as a result of acne, eczema, rashes, smallpox, and other sores or wounds. It is often used to treat herpes outbreaks in the genital area (herpes simplex virus 2).

Berberine found in goldenseal has been studied extensively for its antibiotic effects—especially against bacteria, protozoa, and fungi, as well as candida albicans yeast infections. An overgrowth of yeast and bacteria is often a side effect of taking antibiotics.

Goldenseal contains vitamin C, the B vitamins, vitamin A and E, and the minerals: cobalt, zinc, iron, magnesium, manganese, silicon, calcium and potassium.

Woman should avoid the use of goldenseal during pregnancy, and hypoglycemics should avoid it too as it can lower blood sugar levels.

Hyssop

If you get out your bible and turn to the book of Psalms (51:9) it says "purge me with hyssop and I shall be clean". Hyssop is a Greek word meaning "holy herb"; but cleansing is only one thing that hyssop does.

It is also an excellent antiseptic for treating cold sores caused by the herpes simplex virus, as well as genital herpes. Hyssop is a member of the mint family, and restricts the reproductibe ability of the herpes simplex virus.

It is most effective when used topically as a compress, which can be made by adding 1 ounce of dried hyssop herb to each pint of boiling water. Next, let the mixture steep for 15 minutes and let cool. Then soak a clean cloth in the concoction and apply to cold sores and genital herpes as required.

Licorice Root

Licorice Root has been used for centuries as a treatment for colds, coughs, sore throats, rashes, ulcers, arthritis and colic to name a few. It is also useful for strengthening the adrenal glands and the adrenal cortex.

One of its active ingredients—glycyrrhetinic acid helps reduce the healing time and pain which are linked to cold sores and genital herpes.

Glycyrrhetinic acid irreversibly deactivates the herpes simplex virus and promotes the release of interferon in the body to fight infection. Licorice powder can be applied topically to the affected area to speed up healing.

Various studies have identified its usefulness against various types of viruses including: cytomegalovirus (CMV), Epstein-Barr virus (EBV) and varicella-zoster virus which is responsible for chickenpox and shingles.

Marjoram

Marjoram is often thought of as a spice used in cooking. However, marjoram also has healing properties as well. For a herpes infection, try sprinkling marjoram powder on cold sores and genital herpes to speed up healing. Studies show it restricts the growth of the virus.

Myrrh

We read about myrrh in a biblical sense when the three wise men came to the infant Jesus bearing gifts of gold, frankincense and myrrh. In fact myrrh has been used since around 1550 BC. The ancient Egyptians used it for embalming purposes because of its preserving properties.

Myrrh has excellent astringent, anti-fungal and anti-inflammatory properties and as such, is an effective treatment for a variety of skin problems. Myrrh is an additive in many toothpaste formulas.

Olive Leaf

Olive trees are well known for their resistance to disease, fungal growth and bacteria. Olive leaves have been used for medicinal treatments since the early 1800s.

Olive leaves have been known to eliminate bacterial and viral infections in patients who have been on courses of medication for some period of time without success. In fact olive leaf has been proven to be the first natural treatment which is successful against herpes simplex type 1 (HSV-1) and herpes simplex type 2 (HSV-2) viruses. In fact, olive leaf has proved successful in eliminating all symptoms associated with genital herpes, even where medications have failed to eliminate the problem—such medications as acyclovir, butylated hydroxytoluene (BHT) and the amino acid lysine.

Pau D'Arco

Pau D' Arco or Taheebo to give it its other name is harvested from the bark of the Lapacho tree in South America. Pau D'Arco has been used for centuries by native tribes for a variety of medicinal uses. The bark of the tree is made into a tea and drunk at least three times each day to treat such conditions as dysentery, ulcers and rheumatism.

It is used topically for a variety of skin conditions including: sores, viral infections—especially of the mouth, nose and throat, eczema and snake bite.

It is also used extensively throughout the world as a preventative treatment for cancer.

Peppermint

Peppermint has been used for thousands of year to sooth an upset stomach, and to treat colds, bronchitis and menstrual problems. Peppermint as an oil is a potent agent in killing the herpes simplex virus when applied topically.

Red Clover

Used for over a hundred years by American herbalists to treat inflammatory skin conditions, due to it containing phenolic acids, including salicylic acid. Red clover is also used to treat arthritis, gout, jaundice and liver congestion.

Spirulina

A type of blue-green algae found in fresh water. Spirulina is an excellent source of pre-digested protein, as well as all the 9 essential amino acids in their correct ratios, and trace minerals.

Various studies have been done to prove its effectiveness for many ailments including anemia, cataracts, diabetes a weakened immune system and severe skin outbreaks. Spirulina also has potential to protect the kidneys from damage due to an individual taking strong medications.

St John's Wort

Used for over 2,000 years by herbalists, St John's Wort is used extensively in Germany to treat symptoms of depression. Much research has also been done in Germany and Russia where significant amounts of flavonoids and a substance called hypericin have been found.

Hypericin in St John's Wort is an excellent anti-bacterial, anti-inflammatory and antiviral agent. It is used to treat such conditions as: infections and inflammation.

St John's Wort helps strengthen the nervous system in addition to relaxing muscle spasms and tightening tissue.

Tea Tree Oil

A native of Australia, tea tree oil has proved to be an effective antiseptic against bacteria, fungi and viruses. It is an effective topical treatment for cold sores and herpes infections.

In addition, tea tree oil is also an effective anti-fungal treatment against fungal infections of the skin and mucous membranes.

It is often used in aromatherapy treatments with bergamot, eucalyptus or lavender.

Witch Hazel

I have read some reports that individuals pierce a cold sore and apply witch hazel or alcohol to dry it out. I am not sure whether it works or not, but you might like to consider giving it a try.

Vitamins and Minerals Can Make a Difference Too

Vitamin A

Vitamin A is an antioxidant vitamin and in the case of herpes, it helps boost the immune system and helps reduce a re-occurrence of the infection. However, at high daily doses—above 15,000 international units (IU) for men and 10,000 international units (IU) for women of childbearing age, vitamin A can cause a toxic build-up in the body. It is best therefore to consult your doctor before increase your intake of vitamin A.

Perhaps a safer alternative is to take beta carotene which is a precursor for vitamin A. The body converts beta carotene to vitamin A as it is needed. If it is not needed, then, it is excreted out in the urine.

Vitamin C
Vitamin C—an antioxidant vitamin is well known as being beneficial for helping reduce the effects of the common cold, in addition to boosting the immune system to help fight infections. It is also useful for dealing with cold sores and genital herpes too. At the first signs of an infection appearing—which is usually indicated by a tingling and burning sensation, then taking a high dose of vitamin C with bioflavonoids will lessen the impact, as both these two work together.

So how much vitamin C and bioflavonoids should you to take? 1,000 milligrams of each one is a good amount to start with as soon as the tingling and burning occurs. You could then reduce this to 500 milligrams of each one three times a day and take as required. You can buy 500 milligram and 1,000 milligram tablets of vitamin C, so it is basically just a few tablets—not a whole handful. Some vitamin C supplements contain bioflavonoids as well, but if not, then bioflavonoids can be obtained as a separate supplement.

What are bioflavonoids?
They are a chemical compound which is a close relation to vitamin C. They are basically a group of plant pigments that protect body cells by providing protection as a result of altering the actions of allergens, carcinogens and viruses.

Bioflavonoids give plants and the blossom they produce their color pigments. Bioflavonoids are also found in the white lining which is just under the skin of citrus fruit.

They are also powerful free radical scavengers and help protect the body against the harmful effects of these toxic substances. The body does not produce bioflavonoids therefore they must be obtained from the diet.

Vitamin C is a water soluble vitamin, so it is easily excreted through the urine during periods of stress. If you take too much vitamin C— over 1,200 milligrams a day, then this can cause diarrhea in some individuals. If this happens to you, then just reduce the dose until the diarrhea stops.

Vitamin E

Vitamin E—a powerful antioxidant vitamin is also useful in treating cold sores. Use it topically. Break open the capsules and apply the oil to the blister. It will help to reduce pain and speed up healing. One word of caution! If the cold sore is in your eye area, then consult your physician before applying.

Zinc

Zinc—an antioxidant mineral. It is important for boosting the immune system to help fight infection. It is good too for treating cold sores and genital herpes. Apply an ointment containing zinc oxide directly to the blisters to help dry up the infection and speed up healing.

Women who have vaginal herpes should not use zinc oxide ointment. This is because drying agents should not be used on mucus membranes.

To help in the battle against a herpes infection, you can also supplement with a zinc tablet too—thus attacking the problem from the outside and the inside. How many zinc tablets to take? Supplements usually contain between 15 to 25 milligrams of zinc per tablet, depending on which country you live in. In Europe it is 15 milligrams, in the US 25 milligrams.

The recommendation to fight a herpes infection is anything between 30 to 60 milligrams each day—which is well above the recommended daily amount of 15 milligrams a day. It is best though, to consult your doctor before increasing your zinc intake.

Large amounts of zinc can interrupt the absorption of copper; therefore it is recommended that for every 10 milligrams of zinc, one milligram of copper should be taken.

You can also try zinc lozenges to suck if the cold sore is inside the mouth. Using zinc to treat cold sores can reduce the healing time by anything between 30 to 40 percent.

When purchasing vitamin supplements, always make sure they are from a natural source—not synthetic. Natural vitamins have a life-force which the synthetic ones do not have. Often times the synthetic ones are very cheap, and offers are everywhere of "buy one and get two free", or something similar. Which would you rather put into your body—something that is natural or something that is a chemical spin-off from an industrial process?

Don't Forget the B Vitamins

Although not an antioxidant, the B vitamins play a vital role in maintaining your good health. Like antioxidant vitamins, they help prevent oxidation as well as improving the supply of oxygen to the brain and other areas of the body. They are water soluble so you need them every day as they are easily excreted from the body when it is under stress.

The following is a list of the B vitamins and what they do.

Vitamin B1 (Thiamine)

Thiamine works with other B vitamins to break down food. It functions as a co-enzyme to convert glucose into energy in the muscles, nerves and neurons. It is important for helping the brain use oxygen more efficiently to maintain energy levels, helps to reduce stress or a shingles attack and for good digestion. In addition it assists the body to utilize protein.

Good food sources are: pork, vegetables, milk, cheese, peas, fresh and dried fruit, eggs, wholegrain breads, sunflower seeds, soybeans, brown rice, whole wheat, peanuts and some breakfast cereals.

Vitamin B2 (Riboflavin)

Riboflavin helps maintain the skin, mucous membranes, eyes and the nervous system. It assists in producing steroids and red blood cells and helps the body to absorb iron from food. It is also involved in regenerating the antioxidant glutathione.

You find it in many foods including milk, eggs, breakfast cereals, mushrooms and rice. Riboflavin can be destroyed by ultra violet light so these foods should be kept out of direct sunlight.

Vitamin B3 (Niacin)

Niacin like other vitamins helps convert proteins, fats and carbohydrates into energy as well as keeping the digestive and nervous system healthy. It also helps in balancing blood sugar as well as lowering cholesterol levels. It also operates as a co-factor in cell and neuron respiration. There are two types—nicotinic acid and nicotinamide.

You get niacin in beef, pork, chicken, wheat flour, maize flour, milk and eggs.

Vitamin B5 (Pantothenic Acid)

Pantothenic acid also helps release the energy from food. It is also used by the adrenal glands to produce stress hormones during periods of physical and psychological stress.

Good food sources are: most meats and vegetables especially chicken, beef, potatoes, porridge oats, tomatoes, kidney, eggs, broccoli, whole grains and rice. Some breakfast cereals are fortified with it.

Vitamin B6 (Pyridoxine)

Pyridoxine is necessary for metabolizing the amino acids in proteins, the formation of antibodies and red blood cells, and for maintaining a healthy digestive and nervous system. Vitamin B6 is also needed along with vitamin B12 and folic acid to help lower high homocysteine levels.

Good food sources are: pork, turkey, chicken, bread, cod and whole cereals such as wheat germ, oatmeal and rice. It is also contained in milk, vegetables, eggs, soya milk, peanuts, potatoes and some breakfast cereals.

Vitamin B7 (Biotin)

Biotin is very important in childhood. It helps your body utilize essential fats and is also important for healthy hair, skin and nails. It also helps turn food into energy as well as being involved in amino acid metabolism.

It is found in a great many foods including kidney, egg yoke and some fruit and vegetables, whole grains, and dried mixed fruit.

Vitamin B9 (Folic acid)

Known as folate in its natural form, it works with B12 to form healthy blood cells and helps reduce the risk of defects in babies such as spina bifida. Folic acid is needed along with vitamin B6 and B12 to help lower high homocysteine levels. Folic acid is important for maintaining good brain health and memory, in addition to being a critical component for maintaining a good nervous system

Folic acid is found in small amounts in numerous foods but rich sources are breakfast cereals, some types of bread and fruit such as oranges and bananas. It's also found in broccoli, Brussels sprouts, asparagus, peas, rice and chickpeas.

Vitamin B12 (Cyanocobalamin)

Vitamin B12 helps make red blood cells and generally keeps the nervous system in optimum condition. It helps release energy from the food we eat and it also helps process B9 (folic acid). It deals with the effects of tobacco smoke as well as other toxins in the body. If you don't get enough, you'll probably find that you are anemic. Long term deficiency of B12 can lead to damage of the nervous system, and also an inefficient transport of oxygen to the brain. Vitamin B12 is also needed along with B6 and folic acid to help lower high homocysteine levels.

As we get older it becomes more difficult to absorb B12 through the gut, even though there may be adequate amounts in the diet. In such cases, B12 injections may be recommended.

Vitamin B12 is found in fish, meat, poultry and dairy foods. Since B12 is not found in vegetables, fruits or grains, vegans or vegetarians may find themselves deficient in it.

Vitamin B12 is available in supplement form as part of a Balanced B Complex formula; also B12 can be bought as a stand-alone supplement.

Note. All the B vitamins work together therefore it is best to take a Balanced B Complex supplement. That way you will get all the B vitamins in the correct ratios.

If you need more of a particular B vitamin, then you can take this in addition to the Balanced B Complex supplement. As always, make sure that whatever supplement you take, it is from a natural source–not synthetic.

9. So What is Shingles

Basically it is a herpes zoster virus, or to use its more common name—shingles. Shingles is an infection associated with adults, a bit like chickenpox is associated with children. In fact, both conditions are caused by the same virus.

For some reason, the virus remains dormant within the nerve cells in the body for years, and then suddenly decides—for reasons unknown to reactivate itself as shingles, when the person is a lot older.

The initial sensation of a shingles outbreak is pain or tingling as the virus multiplies as it moves along one of the peripheral nerves that spread outwards from the spine. Interestingly, it only affects the area of your face or body which is served by that particular nerve.

Following the pain and tingling, a rash will appear two or three days later, as the virus finally arrives in the nerve endings in your skin. During the next 3 to 5 days the rash will reach its maximum coverage. This can be identified as rectangular belts on one side of the body extending all the way from the spine to the rest of the body, or on one side of the face or head. The blisters usually dry up in a few days which then form a crust that will eventually fall off in two or three weeks after your initial infection.

Each year around 300,000 Americans have a shingles infection. Although it can occur at any age it is most likely to happen after age 60. A re-occurrence of the infection may happen, but is more likely to do so when you take a medication that suppresses your immune system. If you did not have a chickenpox infection as a child, and later in life you are exposed to the herpes zoster virus, then you will probably have a serious case of chickenpox rather than shingles.

Under normal circumstances shingles is not a serious condition, although it may make life difficult for you as you could possibly continue to have pain for months or even years along the peripheral nerve involved. This condition is called post-herpetic neuralgia and happens in roughly 50 percent of those who have had shingles and are over the age of 60.

It will all depend on which nerve the virus decides to call "home". This will determine which parts of your body will be affected. When the major nerve in your face—the trigeminal nerve is affected the rash can occur on your face and inside your mouth or eye. It is important to understand that any shingles infection in your eye needs immediate medical attention because if it is left untreated, it can lead to permanent damage to your vision.

If you have a weakened immune system, then this can be a real issue if you have shingles; additionally, if you have a HIV infection or are taking chemotherapy drugs for certain forms of cancer such as leukemia and Hodgkin's disease then this can put you at a higher risk of a shingles attack. And finally, any form of transplant surgery where immunosuppressant medications are taken, can also make you susceptible to a shingles attack.

When you do have a shingles attack, it is important not to pick at the blisters as this can spread the infection. Also, you can inflame the skin by applying too many skin creams and ointments. It is therefore best to use these treatments sparingly.

Here is a good preventive tip to help you maintain your good health. It is a good idea to keep away from anyone who has chickenpox, especially if you are feeling under the weather yourself, or if your immune system is impaired, as the chickenpox carrier may trigger an outbreak of shingles in you.

As far as medications are concerned, nothing that you take will shorten the time line of a shingles infection. You can try soaking the blisters with a cool wet compress and then apply a soothing lotion. Taking aspirin, Ibuprofen or Acetaminophen may help reduce the pain of post-herpetic neuralgia.

If you experience a more serious pain and discomfort then stronger painkillers may be needed. Should you have a weak immune system than your physician may prescribe corticosteroids in the early stages of infection to minimize the subsequent neuralgia around your specify infection, or if you have a weakened immune system, and very severe pain then possibly an antiviral agent such as acylovir may prove helpful.

Whilst few medications will have much of an impact on a shingles infection, you may want to look at a few herbal preparations as well as aromatherapy oils, herbal teas and vitamin and minerals supplements. I have described a selection on the following pages.

Medicinal Herbs for Herpes Zoster (Shingles)

Bee Propolis

Honeybees are busy and very industrious little workers. And they are responsible for bee propolis, which is a sticky resin substance gathered by the honeybees from the bark and leaves of deciduous trees. The honey bees use this to seal holes and cracks in their hives.

Here is the neat part! Before the honey bees use it in their hives, they mix the propolis with nectar from their own secretions, and the final result is a mixture of bee bread, pollen and wax.

It has been in use for thousands of years to provide energy and stamina as well as providing protection against the herpes zoster (shingles) virus and to promote healing.

Red Pepper (Cayenne or Capsicum)

This is a real hot one—which owes its healing ability to a chemical found in the fruit called capsaicin. Red pepper or as it is sometimes called: cayenne pepper or capsicum can be applied topically to the skin or mucous membranes. Capsaicin, one of the active compounds in cayenne pepper actually stimulates and then blocks small diameter pain fibers by depleting them of a neurotransmitter called substance P. In studies this neurotransmitter has been identified as activating inflammatory actions in joint tissue.

In studies capsaicin has also been shown to be effective in treating the after pain from a shingles attack known as post herpetic neuralgia. Studies show that the use of a topically applied capsaicin cream is effective in relieving the pain associated with shingles, in cases where the pain has lasted for over 24 months. In the study over half of the people with post herpetic neuralgia responded to a topically applied capsaicin cream. Although this figure does not sound very high, it is a significantly better than the 10 percent improvement achieved by the group taking a placebo.

Capsaicin has been formulated into various Food and Drug Administration (FDA) approved creams. One of these Zostrix is very effective for treating shingles. Zostrix is available as an over-the-counter (OTC) remedy, and is one of the most effective treatments available for the severe chronic pain which often follows a shingles attack.

Oatstraw

Oatstraw is a very useful herb if you still have pain after the attack has subsided. You can use oatstraw as a herbal supplement or as a tincture, which will work best if applied twice daily. Another alternative is to get plenty of oats in the diet, and probably an excellent way of achieving this is to have porridge oats for breakfast. However, instant oats are not always as effective as the proper old-fashioned variety.

Aromatherapy Oils

So far I have hardly mentioned aromatherapy oils in this book. However, they are very useful for treating all forms of herpes. Aromatherapy oils can act as antiviral agents and help reduce pain, as well as drying blisters.

Aromatherapy oils should be diluted with a carrier oil and are best used as combinations of two or three different oils; if a small area of blisters are involved, then it is a good idea to apply the oil on the affected area twice each day; alternatively you can use them in the bath or diluted in water as a warm compress.

Here are three oils to consider: bergamot, eucalyptus and tea tree. Lavender is useful too if pain persists after an infection as it has excellent healing and analgesic properties. Some good combinations to consider are bergamot and tea tree oil, or bergamot and lavender. You can however mix them all together and achieve equal results.

Herbal Teas

Should you feel depressed, after a shingles attack them rosemary is an excellent herbal tonic when made into a tea. Drink a cupful in the morning and then later on in the evening before bedtime, drink a cup of lime blossom tea, which will help you sleep.

Although not an aromatherapy oil or herbal tea here is another couple of ideas for you to consider. If you feel the first signs of an infection, which is best demonstrated by a tingling sensation, then you could try rubbing the affected area with a freshly cut lemon. If you have an attack of shingles a salt bath may bring some relief to help in the healing process and drying of the blisters.

Vitamins for Herpes Zoster Virus

B Complex Vitamins

Taking a vitamin B. complex supplement will help support the nervous system by regenerating and rebuilding nerve cells, as well as helping to reduce stress. The B. vitamins are water soluble and are easily depleted from the body during periods of stress.

Vitamin B1 (thiamine) is particularly useful in helping reduce stress or a shingles attack. Good sources of vitamin B1 include: pork, vegetables, milk, cheese, peas, fresh and dried fruit, eggs, wholegrain breads, sunflower seeds, soybeans, brown rice, whole wheat, peanuts and some breakfast cereals.

The mineral magnesium must also be present in the body in order for thiamine to convert to forms the body can use.

Vitamins B12 (Cyanocobalamin) is also useful in cases of depression and shingles infections. Good food sources of vitamin B12 include liver, organ meats, eggs, dairy products, fish, and meat. Vitamin B12 levels in the body can be depleted by such things as anticoagulant drugs, laxatives, Alcohol, aspirin, antibiotics, caffeine, sleeping pills and contraceptives.

Interestingly, a study by researchers in India have reported that individuals with shingles had a very positive response with regard to relief of pain, and how quickly blisters disappeared after only two or three days treatment with vitamin B12 injections. More importantly, none of these individuals experienced the lingering pain following their shingles attack.

Vitamin B12 injections are more easily absorbed into the body than supplements. Vitamin B12 injections are given by your doctor, either on a daily or weekly basis for a period of several weeks. It is impossible to get large doses of vitamin B12 from foods, however, supplements can be helpful, but it is a vitamin B12 injections, where the highest doses are possible.

Vitamin B12 plays an important role in nerve function. It is needed by nerves to help maintain the protective myelin sheath.

It is important to remember as explained elsewhere in this book that all the B. vitamins work together. It is best therefore to get these in a B. complex form, and then add individual B vitamins as required.

Vitamin C

It is important to look after your body systems. One way you can achieve this is to always ensure that your immune system is operating at peak performance. You can help do this by including a vitamin C supplement as part of your diet. Like the B. vitamins, vitamin C is also water soluble, and is easily depleted during periods of stress. An ideal vitamin C supplement dose would be 1000 milligrams per day. Studies show that in large doses, vitamins C. can restrict the mutation of certain types of viruses, which includes those in the herpes family. Vitamins C. can also restrict the ability of certain viruses to cause infections.

As vitamins C. is an antioxidant vitamin. It has the ability to neutralize inflammation caused by biochemical actions that are produced by immune system cells as they go to work against the shingles virus. This action of vitamins C. may help prevent nearby cells from becoming damaged due to the actions of the immune cells against the virus.

Remember that large doses of vitamins C. can cause diarrhea. The way to remedy this situation is to slightly reduce the vitamins C. intake until the diarrhea ceases.

As mentioned previously in this book, you may also want to consider a vitamin C supplement containing bioflavonoids, or a separate bioflavonoid supplement.

Vitamin E

Vitamin E is another antioxidant vitamin. It helps to protect nearby cells from damage as a result of the immune cells attacking the viral invaders. Vitamin E is a fat soluble vitamin, and as a result is integrated into the fatty membranes of all cells—which includes nerve cells. Nerve cells are protected by the myelin sheath—the thick layer of fatty membranes that wraps around nerves and insulates them.

Multivitamin/Multi-Mineral Supplements

You could also consider taking a multivitamin and a multi-mineral supplement each day to help ensure that you get all the necessary vitamins and minerals your body needs. Multi-vitamins are a good insurance in case of a vitamin or mineral deficiency as a result of a lack of nutrients in the diet.

One of the things about multi-vitamin supplements is that if the body doesn't need any particular vitamin or mineral in the formula, then it will pass out harmlessly in the urine.

Put Together a Supplement Pack for You

It can do no harm, and may do a lot of good by putting together a vitamin and mineral pack for yourself. This will comprise a multivitamin, and multi-mineral supplement, vitamin A. (or its precursor beta carotene), vitamin C and vitamin E. To this you could add the antioxidant minerals selenium and zinc, as well as the essential fatty acids omega-3 and omega 6. This pack will help to support all the body systems, but especially the immune and nervous systems.

As explained elsewhere in this book, always buy natural supplements as opposed to synthetic ones. The synthetic ones may be cheaper, but the natural ones will be more beneficial for you. Ask yourself this, would you rather put a natural element into your body or a synthetic one which has been derived from a chemical base? I know which one I would rather take!

Remember to always eat plenty of fresh fruit and vegetables—especially dark colored vegetables, such as beetroot, cabbage, carrots, broccoli and peppers. All these have excellent antioxidant properties.

You could also include in your diet, grains, white meat such as chicken and turkey, a small amount of red meat and fish—especially oily fish such as salmon, mackerel, tuna and herring. All these fish are excellent sources of essential fatty acids, which must be obtained from the diet as the body cannot manufacture them itself.

In Summary

A herpes virus infection is not very pleasant. And to make matters worse, you have the infection for the rest of your life. The herpes virus seems to be on the increase in the American population, due in part to changes in sexual practices which has meant that the herpes simplex virus type I (HSV-1) which is usually associated with cold sores in and around the mouth, the nose or the eyes, is now being identified in the genital area. And by extension, the herpes simplex virus type 2 (HSV-2) which is normally associated with genital herpes is now being found in the mouth—a place where normally it should not be. This suggests a growing tendency for oral sex and as a result, a mix/match of the herpes simplex virus.

As far as the herpes zoster virus is concerned, or as it is probably better known—shingles, this is a viral disease which mainly affects the elderly, and can cause much pain and distress. What is especially uncomfortable is the severe pain, which in approximately 50 percent of cases follows on from a shingles outbreak. This pain can in some cases last for several months or even years.

It is distressing to know that after so many years, no cure has been found for herpes: either for the herpes simplex virus type 1 or type 2, or the herpes zoster virus. Equally troubling, is that so few medications have been developed to treat the virus.

In this book I have therefore researched quite a few herbal medicines which can bring some relief and comfort to those who are infected with this virus.

I hope that you have found this book useful and that it has given you a better understanding of the virus, whether it is type I, type 2, or the herpes zoster virus. It seems to me that much research still needs to be done in order to find a cure for this virus, either as a vaccine, or better medications.

About The Author

Brian B Jacques started in business at a young age, and over the ensuing years, he has developed several very successful businesses. But his main interest for the past 40 years has been in natural health research and publishing.

Brian has presented seminars worldwide on such diverse subjects as Health Related issues, Motivation and Personal Development. In addition he has written numerous books, newsletters and articles on these subjects.

His very popular series of Mini Health Books has circulated widely around the world, and many more titles are in preparation.

Brian is a highly motivated individual, so much so that in 1985 he received a UK Industrial Society award for his work in the Motivation and Personal Development fields.

Brian has the following mottos:

- If something does not work out for you, then don't give up, but keep trying, trying, trying until finally you succeed.
- Success or failure in any endeavor is in your own hands.

Brian and his wife divide their time between East Yorkshire, UK and Florida, USA.

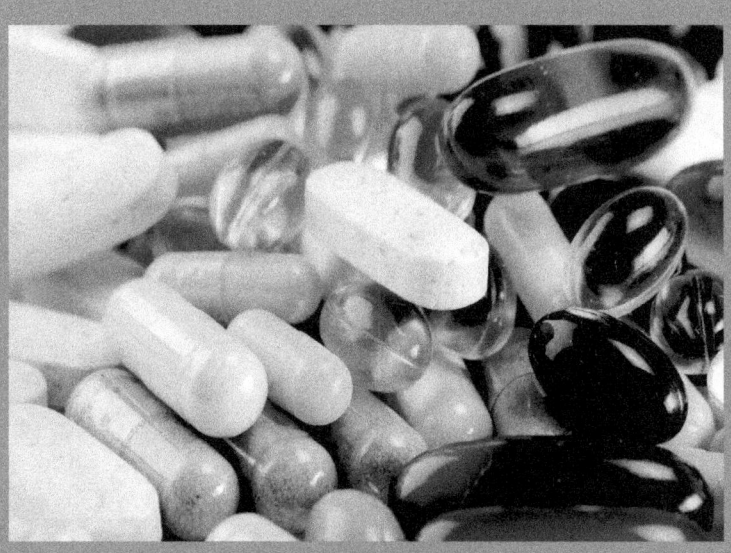

www.ingramcontent.com/pod-product-compliance
Lightning Source LLC
Chambersburg PA
CBHW071249280526
45788CB00004B/1639